NOBODY
NEEDS
TO BE
FAT
ANYMORE!!!

....

One Woman's Fat Life and How She Lost 100 Pounds at Age 70

VIRGINIA KATHLEEN BOYD

Westfeld Press
HUDSON, OHIO

Inquiries to SOS Seminars, Inc., P.O. Box 493
Aurora, Ohio 44202

V.K. Boyd/Westfeld Press
Hudson, Ohio

Book Layout ©2013 BookDesignTemplates.com

Ordering Information:
Quantity sales. Special discounts are available on quantity purchases by corporations, associations, and others. For details, contact the "Special Sales Department" at the address above.

Nobody Needs to Be Fat Anymore/ Virginia Kathleen Boyd -- 1st ed.
ISBN 978-0-9916173-9-5

PREFACE

....

This book is about my fat life and how I LOST over 100 POUNDS *at the age of 70!!*

I didn't starve, I didn't exercise, I wasn't young, and I didn't have gastric bypass surgery. I didn't do most of the things that I had done throughout my life to try to lose weight. It took me learning why I was fat, then learning how to lose weight, and then finally learning how to keep it lost, to win this lifelong battle.

If only I had known when I was young what I know now about food and eating, I might never have had a fat day in my whole life.

During my lifetime, being fat was always difficult. Obesity is the last allowable form of discrimination. Ask anyone who is fat. Fat people are constantly being ridiculed and laughed at, even little kids say the darndest things about fat people.

When my daughter was only seven years old and we were all sitting around the dinner table one evening, I asked her about her new teacher. I wasn't sure that I knew the lady, and when I asked my daughter what she looked like, my daughter piped up and said, "she's fat, even fatter than you mom". Even without realizing it, kids know FAT when they see it too.

We all laughed, and I was a little embarrassed, but honestly, anytime in my life when I was ever confronted about being fat, it didn't change how I felt about myself. You see I already felt good about who I am, and I never allowed my weight to make me feel like less of a good person.

I had grown up in a violent alcoholic home, and back in those days, weight was the least of my problems. But my daughter was right, I was fat.

Like I said, I knew that being fat wasn't all that I am. Despite my weight, I knew that I was still a beautiful person. Not only that, I learned early on in life how *BEAUTIFUL **ALL** PEOPLE ARE*. I learned early that PEOPLE ARE AMAZING. I really mean it!!

If you are a fat kid, or a fat middle aged man or woman or a senior citizen who can hardly get around because you are fat, don't be fooled by the world's arrogance and rudeness. **You are STILL BEAUTIFUL!!**

Just think about it for a minute, PEOPLE ARE AMAZING. We have arms and legs and eyes and ears, things that do things, like see and hear and walk and run. That is all truly amazing! Even if we lose a body part, our other body parts step in to compensate. How incredible is that?

Young or old, rich or poor, we are walking, talking, laughing, and crying miracles and each one of us should feel SO SPECIAL because each one of us **IS SPECIAL**.

Your fingerprint and DNA are yours alone. There will never be another you in the whole world, and at any age, you are a "promise of possibilities", so start off right now by realizing how amazing and special you really are.

Knowing how **SPECIAL YOU ARE** is why I wrote this book. Knowing the struggles of my fat life and how to fix it makes me want to fix everyone else's fat struggles too.

When I see a fat person in a store, or walking down the street, in a restaurant, or anywhere, I watch to see if they struggle to get up, or bend over, or just move around. I almost want to run over and grab them and tell them that I was fat, REALLY fat, and that I finally know how to fix what causes it.

You see, I know how they feel. Even without the extra 100 pounds, I'll always be FAT on the inside, but I never NEED to be fat anymore on the outside, and **NEITHER DO YOU.**

TABLE OF CONTENTS:

CHAPTER ONE

··

FAT BEGINNINGS

I have a younger sister I'll call Penny. Penny is five years younger than me and she was always a skinny kid. I was always jealous of that.

One of my earliest memories of being jealous of Penny's skinny childhood was a visit to the "shaker counter". We lived in a northeast U.S. city, and in the 1950s, the suburbs were just beginning to boom. We lived in the inner city, but our extended family had cottages at a little campsite area in the country about fifty miles away. In the summer, we would travel back and forth to the cottage on a main highway north out of the city.

I remember at first, that the trip was mostly farmland with big red barns and cows standing around on the hillsides. Later the road out of town developed into a major shopping thoroughfare with strip stores, fast food, movie theaters, and malls.

But before all that development came along, the first business that I remember out there was a little store on the front corner of a farm where they sold dairy products.

The place was just a little building that didn't have much glitz, but inside there was a wonderful surprise. They made and sold milkshakes!! We would usually stop there for a milkshake on our way out to the cottage.

On those trips I waited in expectation as we neared the "shaker counter" and that milkshake was the highlight of my cottage trip. Forget about the swimming pool, or the roller rink, or the little carnival that awaited us at our destination at the little park. My big excitement was that milkshake.

The first time I realized that something was different about me and my weight, was at the "shaker counter". My dad came out with milkshakes in white cardboard cups. I remember the cups had a little ivy-ring design around the outside with a cardboard insert on the top which served as a lid. There was a hole on one side of the lid for the straw, and I could hardly wait for my mother to hand me mine as I sat there in the back seat of the car.

My sister shared the back seat with me, and she was also handed a milkshake. We have a brother who is five years older than me, but I can't remember him being there with us on that trip.

I remember sitting behind my mother drinking up the milkshake and looking over at Penny who was playing with her doll. She took a sip of the precious drink, and she leaned the cup against her leg on the seat and went back to playing with her doll.

After a while and after my treat was all gone, I sat there, coveting Penny's milkshake. As my mother kept hounding my sister to finish her drink, I thought about taking it from her, or should I say stealing it from her.

I remember wondering why she was so skinny and why I was so chubby. Why is she never hungry, I remember thinking? I was only about eight or nine years old at the time, but I know that I was secretly jealous that Penny was skinny and wasn't even hungry.

Thankfully, it was soon time to drive away, and my mother told Penny to give her drink to me to keep it from being wasted. Already I was the family "clean-up committee".

While I wasn't really a FAT child, I knew right from those early years that I was wired differently. All the milkshakes at the "shaker counter" wouldn't fill me up. I was ALWAYS hungry, MY WHOLE LIFE!

CHAPTER TWO

....

DIETING UP—WHY FAT PEOPLE STAY FAT

It always surprises me to hear people viciously talk about someone who is fat, like somehow obesity is a crime. I have often heard people ask, "why doesn't she go on a diet and lose that fat" or maybe say things like, "why doesn't she just stop eating"!! Even worse things come out of normally nice people, like calling someone a glutton or a pig behind their back.

I remember one time being out with my husband for a walk along a main roadway in our neighborhood. I was minding my own business walking along on the sidewalk, and someone in a passing car yelled "hey fat a$$" at me out the rear car window. Of course, that behavior told me more about that person's personality than it did about my weight, but it was still embarrassing and frankly astonishing.

What people don't seem to understand about being fat is that fat people DO TRY to lose weight, in fact many times they try, but diets just do not work for most of us.

First off, if someone is fighting a ten or fifteen-pound weight battle, the "metabolism playing field" is still somewhat level and it is possible to shave down that ten pounds through dieting and exercise. It probably doesn't take too long, and most people have the willpower to stay with the regimen long enough to lose ten pounds.

But the fact is that in being fat beyond just a few pounds, it is impossible for us *to stay hungry enough, long enough, to lose enough*© weight, because people DO NOT LOSE WEIGHT by persistent starving. Let me give you an example here of how dieting works for a truly fat person, at least for THIS fat person.

Let's say that I am 225 pounds. I am a 5'6" woman and I am 45 years old. I work in an office, sitting most of the day, but I am running errands and moving around the rest of the time.

I grocery shop and do other shopping while walking all over stores like Walmart and Target. After shopping, I carry in all the groceries, and prepare family meals. Doing laundry, I run up and down stairs from the second floor to the basement. I do dishes and clean up the kitchen each evening. I have two teenagers, and I am a band parent, so I go to football and basketball games on weekends. Mostly I do things, and live a normal everyday life, like people who are not fat.

I have been gaining weight little by little over recent months and even years, and now I realize that since I am getting older and fatter, that I really must do something about my weight, so I decide to start a new diet. Since I have been on diets numerous times before, even achieving my goal weight once, I think I know what to do and what to eat.

I start my diet by eating only about 1400 calories a day. I could try 1200 calories, but at that level, I seem to hibernate, and I begin to store MORE FAT because my body goes into survival mode. It's a really-strange thing that happens when I eat too little and my body thinks I am beginning to starve. Even though I am fat, when I am not eating enough, my body ignores all the fat it could burn, and tries to keep me at my current weight. So, as I begin a new diet, I already know that if I don't eat enough, I won't lose weight either.

Anyway, I have learned that I can lose weight on 1400 calories a day, but that I will gain weight on more than 1800 calories a day. I have a very narrow window of calories between losing and gaining and I can maintain my weight level only at about 1800 calories. So throughout my whole life, when I eat just a little too much, I am gaining weight.

Even just stopping by McDonalds on my way home from shopping or work, and getting a Hot Apple Pie, or a Hamburger might push me over 1800 calories that day and soon my weight will start creeping upwards. While other people are eating those extras, the impact of that little extra food for me is enormous. It seems that I can only maintain my weight when I am perpetually almost dieting.

So now, let's go back to my going on that diet. You might be thinking that I should just stick to that 1400 calories each day and maybe walk off another 100 calories on the treadmill, then I would lose 400-500 calories every day and conquer my weight problem. A pound is 3500 calories, so I should expect to lose close to a pound each week.

That might work, and the Good Lord knows that I have tried that many times before. However, there are several things about that approach that people in the thin world should know about being FAT before they pass judgement on us.

To begin with, FAT people are hungry ALL THE TIME, so cutting back to 1400 calories, and walking on the treadmill for 20-30 minutes a day quickly turns into a daily starvation routine. We wake up hungry and even after each meal, we are still hungry. We go to bed hungry and sometimes wake up in the middle of the night hungry. We are hungry that way even when we are NOT dieting, so it gets even worse when we drop down to only 1400 calories a day.

But fat people are a strong and stubborn breed. We must be strong to endure all the insults, stares, catcalls, and embarrassments in life. So strong are we that we embark on the latest version of our diet with renewed enthusiasm and determination.

As the dieter here, let's see what happens as I begin my new regimen. At 1400 calories and after the first week I may have lost two or three pounds. At my younger age, it might even be four or five pounds. Remembering that most of that loss is the initial water weight, the actual fat loss is probably closer to two pounds of fat. Still it's impressive.

The excitement of seeing that three or four-pound drop on the scale is so stimulating that I commit to "soldier on" for another week. By now though, I am feeling really-really hungry all the time, but my thin friends are telling me to just use my willpower to stay on the diet because it's working.

When I get on the scale at the end of week two, I may have lost another two pounds for a total of five pounds lost, which is encouraging, but I'm still really hungry, and I feel like I have been on this diet for months.

The next week, the end of week three, I get on the scale again and find that I have only lost one more pound, or maybe I didn't lose anything that week. I tell myself that I must be holding too much water weight, or maybe it is because of my monthly cycle, and I plan to have a better loss next week.

By now, however, I have become impossible to live with. I am hungry and angry ALL the time. I resent what other thinner people are eating, and frankly, I become depressed. I never want to go out because everyone "out there" is always eating something, and I cannot give up just yet. By now I have lost a total of six pounds, and that victory was too-hard-fought for me to quit, so I become more isolated and even more hungry.

If I was able to hold out that long, now comes the end of week four. When I get on the scale, I see that I have

GAINED a pound. All those 1400-calorie days, and all the 100 calorie treadmill walks, and all the starving, and all the sacrifice amounts to maybe a loss of five total pounds. I have only gone from 225 pounds down to maybe 220 pounds in a whole month of *sacrifice*.

Now, an onlooker might be saying, "Hooray for you. You lost five pounds!" But I know that the trajectory has shifted. Fat people know what I am talking about. We have ALL done this before. I just GAINED BACK a pound that I fought hard to lose, and next I will be wrestling with losing, gaining or maintaining that pound (or maybe two pounds) for weeks.

Of course, if I continue keeping on my diet, every once-in-a-while the scale will drop an extra pound or two, but by now I am getting discouraged with the small weight loss versus the big **sacrifice,** and I begin to give up.

I was hoping for a steady loss of two pounds a week, totaling at least eight pounds a month. After all, I am try-ing to lose fifty or more total pounds. But here it is, a whole month later, the FIRST and BEST month of weight loss, and I only lost five pounds, and now I have GAINED.

If people wonder why we spend billions of dollars a year on weight clubs, mail order-food, and other diet pro-grams, it is because it takes coercion, either by a coach or trainer or leader, or it takes extravagant spending on food plans to keep us on track. When we stop the diet or the club or the mail-order food, the weight soon piles back on.

But it gets worse. When I finally do give up and begin eating out again, or I eat that Apple Pie or that Hamburger, I almost immediately gain back that first pound or two along with its accompanying water-weight gain. So, in only one week off the diet, I have gained back a pound or two of the weight that it took half a month to lose. Usually though, it doesn't stop there. Like shooting a rubber band, when it snaps back, it sometimes over-shoots.

Our bodies don't have an auto dial that we can reset back to 225, so a week after ending my diet, I get back on the scale and I see that my weight is back up to 223 or 224 pounds and a week later, it is hovering between 225 to 226 pounds. I cannot face the prospect of beginning my starvation regimen again, so I just try to eat on the "low side" and ignore the scale altogether for a while.

But after another month, I hop back on the scale and am crushed to see that I now weigh 229 pounds. After my weight bounces back and forth between 227 and 230 pounds over the next couple of months, I finally land on a new "normal" weight for me at 228.5. Now three or four short months after I started my diet, I am 3.5 pounds heavier than when I began.

Over the years, if I begin my diet once a year with the same result, I will gain 35 pounds in ten years. If I try it twice a year with the same result, I might gain 70 pounds in ten years.

Do you think that's not possible? How do you think people get to be 100 pounds overweight? And as the years go along, we get older and most everything slows down, so the results could be even WORSE.

When normal or thin people ask why FAT people don't diet or why they don't just stop eating, it is because THAT IS HOW WE GOT FAT IN THE FIRST PLACE and why we get FATTER every year!

WE DIETED OUR WAY *UP!!!*

And unlike our normal sisters and brothers, we are hungry and dieting our WHOLE LIVES, and *nothing* we do seems to make us the *same as them*.

CHAPTER THREE

....

FAD DIETS AND OTHER PROGRAMS

My dad was always on a diet. He was an alcoholic, and he had a big beer belly, mostly from drinking lots of beer,. Eventually his drinking killed him, but before that happened, his drinking probably gave him the big belly too. He never wanted to stop the drinking, but he wanted to lose the belly, so he started to fad diet.

Metrical:

The first fad diet that I can ever remember learning about was a powder drink called Metrical. It came in a large can and I think it came in three flavors. I remember the vanilla and chocolate, and there may have been strawberry too. My dad would mix up a Metrical milkshake and drink it two or three times a day and eat a smaller meal once a day.

He did lose a lot of his beer belly, but while it was hardly possible, he was even meaner and angrier than usual, and he only drank the Metrical shakes for about a month. I remember it was during the summer when I was at home and could watch what he did about food each day.

I was only about thirteen or fourteen years old at the time, so it wasn't such a good visual aid for me to see him starving and fad dieting. My weight was already higher than it should have been for someone so young. By the time I was fourteen, I weighed more than 165 pounds, and I was 5'7" tall, so I was already on my way to obesity.

I must have been worried about being fat, because I remember asking my dad if I could have some of the powder to make milkshakes too. That was not a request like at the "shaker counter". I only wanted to try the shakes so I could lose weight. I knew my weight had already climbed out of control and I didn't know what to do to get it back down. I should have only weighed about 140 pounds at that time, so I was already looking at a need to lose around 25 pounds by age fourteen.

I didn't get to try the Metrical though, because my dad yelled at me and told me to leave it alone. He said it was expensive and it wasn't for me. He told me to just stop eating so much, so I never got to try the Metrical. Summer came and went that year without me losing any weight. Soon I was back in school, and my dad had stopped drinking the Metrical shakes and his belly was already getting bigger again.

I was a fairly-ordinary looking girl, so I didn't stand out too much, and being overweight wasn't much of a problem. I was just self-conscious about not being thin like some of the other kids. Of course, kids that age all have problems with body image what with skin problems, and hair styles, and boys getting their facial hair and their voices changing, so nobody at school was really very concerned about my weight. At least nobody bothered me about it.

By the next summer, I had outgrown the clothes that my mother had bought me for school the year before. I was up to 175 pounds then, and I had a straight skirt and blouse, something that you would call a pencil skirt today, and by then I could hardly zip up the side zipper of the skirt. Once when my dad saw me in it, he yelled at me and told me I was getting a fat a$$ and that I should lay off the groceries. I was only fifteen at the time.

Eggs and Grapefruit Diet:

I soon thought that it was lucky for me that it was another summer and another fad diet season for my dad. This year, the Metrical diet was "**out**", and the eggs-and-grapefruit diet was "**in**".

My dad bought grapefruit in big twenty pound mesh bags, and because there were lots of grapefruits, he didn't mind me taking a couple of them each day. He also bought big cans of grapefruit juice and some peeled canned grapefruit which were all off-limits to me because the canned fruit was expensive. But the grapefruits were okay for me to take.

His eggs-and-grapefruit diet was typed on a one-page piece of paper, so I picked it up one day and copied the whole diet into my school notebook. I wanted to write it down for myself so that in case he put it away or it disappeared, I would still know how it worked. THIS WAS MY FIRST FAD DIET.

I wish I knew then what I know now about losing weight because I might NEVER have been fat my whole life. But I didn't know then what I know now, and instead I just mistakenly stumbled into fad dieting.

I did follow the eggs and grapefruit diet most of that summer. I was eating scrambled eggs and half-grapefruits for almost every meal. The grapefruits were sour, but my dad had bought a sugar substitute called cyclamate which I used to sweeten the grapefruit. Cyclamate is now banned in the United States, but it was common at that time.

I followed the eggs-and-grapefruit diet diligently from the middle of June to the middle of August and I lost about 20 pounds. I also went downstairs to our basement game room and exercised on the tile floor in between every meal that summer.

It was the summer between my sophomore and junior years of high school, so when I went back to school in my junior year, my weight was closer to what it should have been for my height and age. Also, my dad stopped insulting me all the time about being fat.

I thought I had done a good thing losing that weight. I began to make all my own clothes on my grandmother's old sewing machine. My weight loss and my more grown-up clothes made me look better as I got older.

After high school, I went to work in a large corporation. It was a good job and I finally had money to buy some clothes and some food that I liked, but my weight began to creep back up again. I panicked about gaining back my weight, so I tried to follow the eggs-and-grapefruit diet once more, but it didn't seem to work again. It might have been because I wasn't exercising between each meal, or that I was eating other things during the day besides eggs and grapefruit. I did try it a couple of other times in my life, but it never worked for me again.

Aids Candies:

Back in the 1960s before the HIV virus came along, there was a diet supplement called Aids Candies. They were little one-inch caramel squares individually wrapped. They came in a box of about thirty candies, and the idea was that if you chewed up a couple of the candies before each meal along with a hot drink like tea or coffee, that you would feel less hungry when it was time to eat and that you would eat less.

Since the eggs-and-grapefruit diet wasn't working anymore, and my weight was back up near 160 pounds, I knew that I had to do something. Of course, my dad was already on the Aids Candies diet, so there were candies around, but I didn't dare take his fad diet candies. I had tried everything that he had tried, except being an alcoholic, but I wasn't welcome to take his diet supplements. So one day, on my lunch hour in town, I bought a box of the candies and tried them out for myself.

I'm not exactly sure if I did the candy diet right or not, but I was honestly never any less hungry before meals and in fact, I would have liked to have eaten a whole handful of the candies at once.

I don't like caramel, but they also came in chocolate, and I loved those. I probably went though the box of candies in less than a week, and they didn't help me to lose weight. Of course, I didn't see much improvement in my dad either, so I don't think that diet idea really worked well, at least as much as I could tell.

During those early adult years, as time went along, I mostly just ate smaller portions or skipped meals, or drank lots of tea and coffee, anything to keep from getting fatter. I really didn't know how to eat healthy, and I never really understood why I was always struggling with my weight since I didn't see everyone else struggling too.

Even though I was working, I only had so much of a budget to work with, so I knew I had to keep my weight within ten pounds of when I had bought or made my clothes. I really couldn't afford to replace clothes for work, and I didn't want to get fatter either.

Weight Watchers–Early Years

While Weight Watchers is basically a sound and healthy program, during the early years the program was sometimes hard for me to follow. I first joined Weight Watchers in 1972 soon after the birth of my oldest child, and since then, I have probably rejoined the program at least fifteen or twenty times over more than 40 years.

When I went into labor with my first baby, I topped out at 197 pounds, and then only dropped 10 or 15 pounds after his birth. I knew I had to do something to lose weight, and my brother's wife had joined Weight Watchers, and recommended it to me. I joined up and after following the program for a few months, I did get my weight down to 170 pounds, but then I got discouraged and finally dropped out without reaching goal.

Weight Watchers was a new approach to weight loss back in those days, and while it did help me to learn and to understand more about food than I ever knew before, it was a fairly-rigid program. In those early days, there were few food options and there were also some required foods like fish, which I didn't know how to make, and liver which I didn't like.

After quitting Weight Watchers, my weight began to creep back up again, and when I had my second child twenty-seven months after the first, I weighed 215 pounds by the time I went into labor. I only dropped to around 200 pounds after her birth, and from there, my weight problem was a constant up-and-down yo-yo for years afterward.

I tried my fad diets again, and joined Weight Watchers several more times, but still I couldn't overcome the constant cycle of losing and regaining weight each time.

Finally, there was a time in 1983 when I rejoined Weight Watchers and I reached my goal weight of 140. To reach that goal, I had stayed on the program for more than nine months, and I walked three miles around my neighborhood every day after work.

It was still hard to follow the program since there were a limited number of exchanges, and I was eating the same foods almost every day. Also, I was tired of feeling deprived all the time. I was always hungry and since I was never a good cook, I ate a very limited variety of meals for all those months. But it was the lowest my weight had been since high school, and I was very thankful that the program worked for me that time.

At first, I did maintain my weight for a while, but I never completed my six weeks of maintenance and I never started my lifetime membership. After a couple of years, some serious personal problems cropped up, and soon I lost interest in worrying about my weight all the time.

As the years went along, my clothes got tighter and tighter, and I kept buying bigger and bigger clothes until I was more than 100 pounds over-weight.

I did rejoin Weight Watchers many times, especially when I worked for a large corporation that had the Weight Watchers at Work program. I probably rejoined every year in January for at least ten years, but by February or March, my losses were small, and my hunger was large, and I soon became discouraged and would quit.

I didn't give up on Weight Watchers though, and years later it helped me to succeed in finally learning what REALLY WORKS in losing weight.

More on that in a later chapter of this book.

Nutrisystem:

I never really followed the Nutrisystem program, but I did sign up for it and I did receive my first one-month supply of food. When it arrived, I opened the box up, and read the instructions, and looked over the food selections, and quickly realized that it would not work for me.

It seemed like there were lots of packets of powdered shakes, and packages that looked a bit like candy bars, and from remembering the old Metrical shakes that my dad drank, I decided that the program wasn't right for me.

I bundled everything up and sent it back for my full refund. I think I needed to pay for the return shipping, but I decided to lose the money in sending it back since everything was brand new and it all might work for someone else.

I did work with a lady a few years later who also tried Nutrisystem, and it didn't seem to work for her either. She had a thyroid condition and was becoming diabetic, and she was always trying to keep her weight under control.

I didn't know that my colleague was trying Nutrisystem until one day she walked in with a big cardboard box filled with Nutrisystem products, and she set it under her work table. She then sent out an email to everyone in the department telling us that she had a box of Nutrisystem food, and if anyone wanted some, they were welcome to come and help themselves. I don't think it was right for her either.

Jenny Craig:

Back when I joined Jenny Craig, Jenny was still very much engaged in the organization and was making membership tapes and doing commercials. I opted for the lifetime membership program, and I received a couple of boxes of her recorded tapes to watch at home and a big binder with lots of information about the program. I was excited about the prospect of trying something new that I hoped would work.

I used to go to the Jenny Craig Center on Monday evenings after work, and at first, I met with a very helpful counselor each week who weighed me and offered encouragement before she took my food order for the next week. Then she went back to the freezers where she helped the receptionist pack up my food for me to take along for the next week, after I paid for my purchase.

Back then it cost me around $100 to $125 a week but that did not include the cost of all the other food I ate

every week. I still had to purchase all my fruits and vegetables and dairy and some other foods. So, at $400 to $500
a month for the Monday purchases, it was a big item in
my budget.

Like all the other diets I ever tried, at first things were
going well and I was losing weight. Most weeks I was losing a couple of pounds for the first month or two, but
then things began to slow down.

I think I stayed with the program for less than six
months and I lost maybe 20 to 25 pounds, I can't remember exactly. It wasn't more than a month or two after I
joined though, that my counselor left. From then on, I had
a series of other fill-in people who mostly just weighed
me and took my food order and sent me off with my purchases every week.

By the fourth or fifth month I was discouraged, and
the weekly cost for my Monday food was beginning to
"bite" too. Each Monday when they tallied up the cost of
my order, I always wrote a personal check to cover the
purchase.

One Friday I was sitting at my desk at work when the
phone rang, and it was the receptionist at Jenny Craig asking me to stop in after work to pay for the food that I had
purchased the previous Monday. I told her that I had already paid by check, and she told me they didn't have my
check anymore, and that they needed my payment.

I questioned her about what happened to my check until she finally told me that the center had been robbed
overnight on the previous Monday night and the check

was gone. They had reported it to the police, but they probably wouldn't be able to get the check back.

I almost imploded when I learned that my check was stolen back on Monday night and now it was Friday when I was finally hearing about it. If I had known right away that my check had been stolen, I would have immediately stopped payment on it, and gone to their center to pay my bill again.

It wasn't just that I was upset that they needed another check. If my first check had gotten lost in their things or been somehow destroyed, I would have totally understood. I was alarmed, however, that some thief somewhere had my check for almost a whole business week, and nobody notified me in all that time.

I did stop in after work that day, and I paid Monday's bill with my credit card. Soon after that, because I was discouraged about both my slow weight loss and about the robbery, I stopped going to Jenny Craig altogether.

Gastric By-Pass Surgery:

I didn't go through with gastric by-pass surgery, but I did sign up to begin the process of getting approved to have the operation. I remember showing up one day at the desk of a nearby hospital for my appointment to attend their in-person seminar on bariatric by-pass surgery. I signed the register and went into the waiting room with the other surgery candidates.

We were all pretty fat, but while I could tell that I was as fat as everyone else, I somehow didn't think I should be there. But lately, I had been thinking that I was on my way to 300 pounds, and I was becoming desperate to get my weight under control.

At that time, I worked with some women who had had gastric by-pass surgery and they seemed to lose a lot of weight fast, although I think one of them was gaining some back. Anyway, I didn't think any of them ever got what I would consider thin, or even what I thought was near a Weight-Watchers type goal, but I still thought they had lost a lot of weight and I decided that I might try it too.

That day at the hospital was very uncomfortable for me. The problem mostly was that all the speakers were telling us how serious the surgery was, and how many ways it would change our bodies and our lives. It seemed like they were trying to discourage us from having the operation.

I also hadn't realized that there were different surgery options, none of which I really understood, so that was confusing me too. Then there was a huge process involved to get approval from our insurance companies, so this was just the beginning of what seemed to me to be a big ordeal. For me, it was a very scary day, and I almost got up and left.

After everyone was done speaking, I pliantly followed the herd and signed up to schedule a meeting with a counselor for later. I would need to have ongoing meetings with my counselor, and I think I also needed to start some sort of a diet. It could have taken as much as six months before I would have the surgery. That would be more than enough time for me to back out, which I did within only a couple of weeks.

I might have met once with my counselor–I can't remember anymore–and I do remember rounding up documentation about all my previous efforts to lose weight. Finally, though, I just called up the hospital one day and cancelled my next counselling appointment, and that was the end of that for me on gastric by-pass surgery. I would need to think of something else.

All My Attempts to Lose Weight:

There were other attempts and ways that I tried to lose weight, and as anyone can tell, I am a veteran FAT person and serial-dieter. By now, I should be in the Dieting Hall of Fame. Unfortunately, all those unsuccessful fad diets and weight loss attempts have chased me through most of my life–my FAT LIFE.

The questions that have always troubled me most are "Why did I always tend to gain so much weight in the first place?" and "Where did my weight problem begin anyway?"

CHAPTER FOUR

....

GROWING UP FAT

So how exactly did I get so fat, and where did it begin? Of course, genetics plays a part in how our bodies work. Just look at the difference between my sister and me. She took after my mother and I took after my dad. Because of that, I thought being fat was my God-given destiny. I used to think that when God was handing out fat cells, that I got a double or triple serving of them.

But when I FINALLY LEARNED what works, I can look back and clearly see what didn't work. As it turns out, it is **ALL ABOUT THE FOOD**. I know now that it wasn't about my age because I have lost more than 100 pounds at the age of 70.

It wasn't about my activity either. While activity is good for our bodies, and I might have lost weight faster had I been more active, what I was doing while I was losing more than 100 pounds, is mostly sitting in the same spot at the one end of my sofa.

Well then, maybe the reason I was so fat was that I was just eating too much. No, it wasn't food volume either.

Remember, I was on diets most of my life. I probably ate less than other people most of the time I was getting fat.

No, for me it was none of the above. What really happened for me was that when I finally learned what works, I lost weight eating enough food to keep me from being hungry all the time. I ate foods that I wanted, whenever I wanted, and in some cases, as much as I wanted, but the KEY was that I was eating DIFFERENT and better foods. So, let's go back to my childhood to see how it all started for me.

My mother was not a good cook. My father used to call her "high-burner Helen". She fried everything over a high gas flame, and she used lots of shortening. She threw burgers, pork chops, sausage, any meat right into the skillet along with the shortening, and soon it was sizzling and splattering. The chicken was always fried, and the breading was always saturated in fat too. I didn't know there was any other way to cook meat.

She also cooked lots of carbs. Every day, there were always foods like mashed potatoes, or macaroni and cheese, or buttered noodles served with what she called "supper". When she made mashed potatoes, she didn't just peel a potato for each of the five of us. No, she peeled the whole five-pound bag of potatoes. She cooked them up and then mashed them, with lots of milk and butter, with her electric mixer.

I remember that she had a set of four glass serving bowls. Each bowl was a different size and color and the biggest bowl was yellow. The yellow bowl was at least a gallon in size, and she would fill that bowl with mashed potatoes, pile it above the top really, and it would sit majestically right in the middle of the table for the five of us to eat.

Then she would open a 12-ounce can of green beans and cook them up too. She would set the small bowl of green beans on the table right there next to the big bowl of mashed potatoes and whatever meat she had fried up that day. Didn't she realize that the big bowl should have had green vegetables, and the small bowl the potatoes?

It didn't matter how many mashed potatoes she made though, because she expected there to be left-overs and she knew a trick on how to fry them too. She would put the big bowl with any leftovers into the refrigerator, and the next evening, she would take out the bowl of cold potatoes and squish them into patties like she was making thick hamburger patties. She would then drop those potato patties into her hot shortening and fry the patties until they were crispy brown on both sides. They were delicious and were probably about 500 calories each.

Nobody else in the family has ever been able to replicate those potato patties. When anyone else tries it, the potatoes dissolve in the skillet into one big potato mess. She died in 1988 and isn't here to tell us what she put into those potatoes when she originally whipped them up that made them stick together in the hot grease. It's probably better that we don't know anyway.

She was the same with macaroni and cheese. She would cook up a pound or two of elbow macaroni and slice off a big hunk of Velveeta cheese from the two-pound block, and add milk, and cook the cheese into the macaroni until it bubbled. She probably used a quarter of the block of Velveeta each time she made the mac and cheese for dinner.

Of course, her buttered noodles and spaghetti were the same way. Lots of carbs, swimming in butter or cheese or sauce. And somehow, she didn't get fat.

She was only about five-feet tall, and she weighed less than a hundred pounds when she got married. Most of my childhood she was closer to 125 pounds, and later in life she was closer to 150, but throughout my early years, she wasn't what I would ever call fat.

The other thing my mother liked was desserts. She didn't make small things like cookies or lite things like Jello. Mostly she baked cakes. She would bake a round two-layer cake and ice it in between the layers and all around, making sure the last of the frosting was piled on the top. Her slices weren't small either. Anyway, there was usually a cake around someplace. Of course, there were big glasses of milk, and bread and butter, always too much fattening food. We had lots of serious problems in our home but going without high-carb food wasn't one of them.

Looking at food and what my family and I ate, it is easy to see how I got off track so early. Maybe for some kids, it doesn't matter what foods are served at home, since some kids might not have such a tendency towards gaining weight, but far too many kids today are fat, and even more are headed that way.

Kids mostly eat what they're fed, so growing up eating fat food often leads to fat children and then onto a new generation of fat adults. Kids don't have much control over what groceries are bought at the supermarket or what foods are cooked in the kitchen. Kids live with the choices their parents make, and when it comes to food, mostly the choices are their mother's. I think that is what happened to me, and that is where and how my lifelong battle with fat all began.

CHAPTER FIVE

....

BRUTALLY TREATED AND
ABUSED

Because I grew up in an alcoholic home with lots of problems associated with anger and violence, I learned early to be strong, and resilient. That is why I never much cared what anyone thought about me or about my weight.

I learned to like myself for the person I am, and it didn't matter whether a diet had worked, and I was smaller or whether I had gained 100 pounds and I was enormous. I always thought that God loved me and that I was a worthwhile human being.

The one thing I didn't like though, was watching others being mistreated because of their weight, or because of any other differences they might have.

I remember one afternoon while I was working at my first corporate job. It was the home office of a national corporation, and I worked in the executive building. It was a twelve-story building downtown, and I took the city bus each day into town and walked all the way across town to my office there. In those days, I was fairly-lean from walking all over town to get to and from work, and from going out most lunchtimes walking around too.

During the workday, I had a fifteen-minute coffee break in the middle of the morning and again in the middle of the afternoon. I was not an exempt employee at the time and breaks were standard procedure for most employees. Usually at break time, a couple of us girls would hop on the elevators and head down to the coffee shop next to the lobby.

On one July afternoon, my regular coffee-break friends weren't available to go down with me at break time, so I decided to go down and bring up a soda to drink at my desk. Just before the elevator doors closed, a couple of girls from another department hopped on with me for the ride down.

Both girls were friendly and chatty, and one of them invited me to join them at the coffee shop. I didn't really know them, but since I am a bit of an introvert and not prone to making lots of new friends, I decided to join them for my break.

In the coffee shop, we slid into an empty booth, and I ordered my soda and I can't remember what they ordered, but soon the talk turned to the beautiful hot summer day it was out there. It must have been a Friday because they were sitting there discussing their summer plans for that weekend. I sat there and sipped my soda as they began talking about how they were going to the swimming pool, and how they could sunbathe and watch all the fat people in their swimming suits.

They were laughing and joking about how ugly the fat girls looked in a bikini and how much fun they would have at the pool. They were so engaged in making their plans, that they hardly noticed that I was even still there with them. It's a good thing too, because my eyes were probably as big as saucers at the shock of hearing them ridiculing other people like that right in front of me.

As I sat there listening in amazement, I thought to myself that they must not know that I am really a fat person. To them, I must have looked like just any other thin person, but I am really a fat person inside. Just then I realized that on the inside, I will really be a fat person all the rest of my life and for that, I will always be thankful.

After I recovered a bit from my shock, I finished up the last of my soda and thanked them for the invitation and excused myself back to work. I never joined them again for a coffee break, and I really didn't see them often, but when I did run across either of them, I was reminded of how hurtful people can be to others who are different.

As I got older, I realized that the ridiculing didn't stop behind peoples' backs either. Sometimes people are mean and cruel right to our faces.

Later, when I was pregnant with my first child, I was gaining weight faster than recommended. My husband and I were young and poor. We got married when he was still in the Marine Corps and my unplanned pregnancy began about a month before his enlistment ended. In his new job, my pregnancy was a pre-existing condition, and wasn't covered by his company's health insurance so the whole pregnancy was a stressful time both physically and financially.

My doctor was a well-known and highly-respected obstetrics doctor who had treated other members of my family. He had treated my mother, and he had delivered my niece and nephews. My grandfather died during my pregnancy, and he had left me $250 which was just enough to pay for the doctor's services, but we ended up owing more than $2,000 for the hospital. Figuring out how to pay that upcoming bill was higher on my list of worries than my being on a diet.

Each month I went in for my regular monthly doctor checkups until about month six when the doctor began to scold me about my weight gains and decided to start seeing me more often. I had already gained 15 or 20 pounds and he seemed to think that I had gained almost enough weight for the ENTIRE pregnancy. He insisted that I return in two weeks, and he warned me not to gain more weight before then.

Two weeks later I returned for my two-week follow-up exam, and I sat on one of the chairs that were lined up along the corridor outside of the three examining rooms. Sitting there, it was always easy to hear the discussions going on between the doctor and his patient in the exam rooms, as well as hearing the nurses who were always going in and out of the rooms.

Finally, it was my turn to be seen. I hopped on the scale, and it showed that I had a three-pound gain. The nurse kind of groaned when she saw my weight gain, and I turned a little sick inside too. That day I also had to give a blood sample, and it was always almost impossible to get blood out of me. My veins are deep, and they roll away when poked. I have the universal blood type and can give blood to anybody, but I could never give blood at the bloodmobile because it is too hard to get it out of me.

After my being both jabbed at and discouraged about my weight gain, the doctor finally came into the examining room carrying my chart. I could see by the scowl on his face that he was annoyed–almost angry–but even I couldn't imagine how brutal it was going to be.

First, he told me that he saw that I had another big weight gain. He reminded me that I wasn't supposed to gain more weight from two weeks ago. I told him that I was sorry, but apparently, I wasn't penitent enough because he stood there and firmly planted both feet on the floor as he faced me directly and began to say that "he didn't care how I *looked* because he didn't have to walk down the street with me", and "he didn't care how *fat I got* because he didn't have to buy my clothes".

But he said that "he would need to deliver this baby and if he was going to have a safe delivery, and if I wanted to have a healthy baby, that I was going to have to control my eating and my weight."

When his tirade had gotten as far as "walking down the street with me", I began to cry, and snot was running from my nose. Without him even looking back, he reached around his side to the counter behind him and picked up the box of Kleenex and held it in front of me as he went on about "not having to buy my clothes". I took some Kleenex and blew my nose and wiped my eyes as he continued to scold me. When he finished his lecture, he told me to come back in two more weeks and he stomped out.

I sat there stunned. I didn't think three pounds was that big of a deal, but then the nurse came in to help me get my things together and as I sat on the table wiping my nose and eyes, she apologized to me for his behavior. She said that she could hear him from the hallway, as I knew everyone could, and she told me that he had lost a new mother that day. She said that his patient had taken her new baby home, and she had two older toddlers. It must have been too much for her and she hemorrhaged and died.

The nurse said he was just upset over his patient, and I felt bad about that. But I also felt like he thought I was as big as an elephant. As I left the room, I could see five or six other women sitting on the chairs in the hallway, waiting their turns to see the doctor. I could tell they felt bad for me, and I was embarrassed about my weight.

I wasn't the only patient that this doctor ridiculed. My brother's wife also went to him for all her pregnancies. One summer, she went in for one of her pregnancy check-ups and she also gained more weight than he approved. He asked her what she had been eating, and she told him they had a cookout. She said that she had eaten a small steak, and a salad, and some corn on the cob. He snapped at her too, as he told her that "corn was for slopping hogs". Naturally, she was humiliated.

Almost everyone who went to this doctor was afraid of him. It was hard to tolerate his fat abuse, but he was a great doctor, and someone that women would stand in line to see. Of course, he probably didn't have an ounce of fat on him.

He was tall and thin and in his early 50s. Up until then, he had never been married, since being a doctor was his life. His father had been an obstetrician before him, and he probably inherited the practice from his dad. He mostly lived at the hospital, but a couple years after the birth of my son, he finally married a widow with grown children. Hopefully, she helped take the edge off his corrosive bedside manner.

There are many other stories I could tell about mean insults towards fat people. It is common to see people staring at obese others walking by, or to see people smiling or rolling their eyes towards someone who is hobbling or waddling along.

It is interesting that many lean people are destined one day to learn how difficult it is to lose weight since most people fill out as they get older. It is said that death and aging are two of the great equalizers, and every second, we inch closer to both.

I don't wish obesity on anyone, but when naturally lean people start to age, they often begin to battle their own expanding waistlines. Those of us who have fought that war early and often, are thankful that we have developed eating and coping skills that have served us well.

By the way, my doctor was a GREAT obstetrician, but he didn't know *anything* about corn. More on that later.

CHAPTER SIX

....

MY REALLY FAT YEARS

W hen my children were teenagers, we moved to a new city where I had to find a new job and was facing all of the pressures of the 40's years and beyond.

I had lost a lot of weight in my mid 30's, and had even reached my goal weight, but due to personal issues and inattention to the scale, my weight had slowly begun to creep back up. Over the next seven or eight years, I gained back more than half of the weight I had lost, and now I was entering menopause. Here then was a new challenge that I hadn't planned on or anticipated, and ultimately it had a BIG impact on my weight.

During my late 40's, I began having more-frequent, longer, and heavier periods, and my clothes were fitting ever-so-much tighter. Since I had moved to a new city several years earlier, I had to sign up with a new doctor, and I picked someone close to my home there. As my yearly check-ups came and went, I noticed that I was having new and increasingly more serious female problems to report at each visit, and I was complaining to my doctor more and more about my monthly cycle.

Finally, my periods got so heavy that I was having trouble keeping up with my normal work and home schedule during at least one week out of every three or four. I soon had multiple appointments with my doctor, to try to resolve my condition, and I took his advice and took any medications he prescribed, but things kept getting worse.

At my last visit with him, my doctor seemed so totally dismissive about my frequent complaints, that I was beginning to self-diagnose, and I finally decided to just tell him that I needed to have a hysterectomy. When I said the word, he reared up like I had touched a nerve, and by my even saying the word "hysterectomy", I felt that I had wandered into some forbidden doctor "inner sanctum". After he regained his composure, he brushed off my hysterectomy request as though I was just being silly. I thought he was much less concerned about me than my previous doctor who had fat-shamed me, and I wasn't sure who I disliked more.

Not long after that last visit, I had gone out from work to the mall at lunchtime, and as I drove back to the office, I started my period in the car and was soon sitting in a puddle in the driver's seat. I didn't even bother to return to work since I would have walked back into the office dripping from my skirt, so instead I just drove straight home for the rest of the day.

Hemorrhaging like that reminded me of when I was a teenager. Back then, I once woke up in the middle of the night, and opened my bedroom door, and there was my uncle Howard in the hallway mopping our hardwood floors. Uncle Howard was my mother's brother and he lived with my aunt and cousins in his house next door. I didn't often see him around, but here he was mopping our floors in the middle of the night.

It seemed that my mother had hemorrhaged, and she was taken away to the hospital in the wee hours of the morning without me even waking up in all the hubbub. And here now was Uncle Howard who had been recruited to clean up the mess that was left behind. My mother had a hysterectomy right after that night, and she returned home again in a couple of weeks.

That day when I hemorrhaged and went straight home at lunchtime, I had the memory of my mother's experience weighing heavily on my mind when I decided to put in an immediate call to my doctor. I thought that he surely would now order surgery just to keep me from being carted off in the middle of the night too.

When he finally returned my call, and I explained what had happened to me that day, his response was his usual "wait-and-see" reaction. I guess he thought I would either get too old to have periods anymore or I would just die off sometime. Either way he didn't seem concerned, and his reaction totally frustrated me. I was feeling frantic as I again pleaded for a hysterectomy, and I was astonished as he brusquely told me that doctors don't do hysterectomies anymore because it is too radical a procedure *just for hemorrhaging*.

That was the wrong thing to say to me, and those were the last words that I ever allowed him to say to me. My "back went up" as I told him in no uncertain terms that if the MEN doctors, and the MEN who ran insurance companies, were gushing blood from their penises, that they would immediately approve ANY and ALL operations that would fix the problem, but because my problem was only a "female problem" and I was just a "silly dumb woman", that I should be ashamed to even ask for a hysterectomy. Then I slammed down the phone, and I never spoke with him again.

In those days, my husband had different medical insurance than I had, and his was a PPO, so I called and scheduled an appointment with a doctor through his insurance at his nearest PPO clinic for as soon as I could get in to see someone. When I finally got to my first appointment with my newest doctor, I was having worse problems with my periods, and she recommended that I go on hormone replacement therapy. I didn't really know what HRT was, but I was so desperate to have something help fix my escalating condition that I quickly signed up for treatment.

Before I left that PPO clinic that day, I had my first prescription of HRT and was on my way to becoming FATTER THAN EVER.

I still don't really understand what the hormones did, except that they did NOT improve my condition. I was still suffering with heavy periods which were only getting worse. I wore only very dark colored clothes and brought my lunch to work every day so that I would not be out and away from the bathrooms. I also tried to keep my meetings at work shorter so I could run to the bathroom more often as needed.

I kept taking the medication, and after about six weeks, my clothes were fitting tighter. I had some loose dresses, and other loose-fitting slacks to wear to work, but after another month or two, I was even bursting out of my fatter clothes. After about five months on the HRT, I made another appointment to go back to my newest doctor, and when I got in to see her and got weighed again, I found that I had GAINED ALMOST 40 POUNDS in five months.

Not only that, but I had almost turned into a maniac too. It was like having PMS all the time, for FIVE WHOLE MONTHS. I don't think I even realized how fat I had gotten while living in the fog of feeling pre-menstrual ALL THE TIME. Things had gone from bad to worse since I still had my original miserable problem, and now I was 40 pounds heavier, AND a *nervous wreck*.

At that visit, I told the doctor that I wouldn't take the medication anymore, and that she would need to try something else to fix my problem. I also asked her about having a hysterectomy, but she didn't even respond to my request. She told me to climb on the table while she "took a look". She had a nurse come in and sort of hold me down while she probed around inside and finally did something that really HURT. Whatever she did, took my breath away, and I could hardly get back on my feet when she finished.

The nurse gave me some supplies to get me dressed and out the door, and as I drove home, I was feeling a little sick and faint all the way. When I got out of the car in my driveway, I could only hobble in the door, and as I glanced down the hallway to the kitchen where everyone else was waiting for me with dinner, I just limped directly up the steps, changed into a robe, and fell into bed. I don't think I moved from the spot until the next morning, and when I got up, I felt SO MUCH BETTER.

To this day, I don't know what that doctor did. Knowing more about female conditions now than I did then, I think it must have been an ablation or a cauterization of some kind. I can't remember if I ever went back to that doctor again, but the previous doctor was right. I did not need a hysterectomy, but he didn't fix the problem either. The second doctor fixed the problem but gave me a NEW problem. I WAS ANOTHER 40 POUNDS FATTER.

By then I was about 60 or 70 pounds overweight. I was almost 50 years old and after that, menopause was a cinch, but from there, my weight turned out to be my biggest physical hurdle.

By then, I had changed jobs to another company where I worked for the next twenty years. After I was at my new company for about three years, my husband's manager came to work at the same company as me and soon recruited my husband to come there too. I didn't love having my husband work at the same company as me, but it was a big place with many buildings, so we didn't see each other often at work.

What we did do however, was we rode to work together. We would go to my building first where he dropped me off, and then he would park at his building for the day and do the reverse at the end of the day when it was time to pick me back up.

Lunches were the other thing we did the same, and **lunches is where I think I gained the rest of my weight.** I never understood why I kept gaining weight all the time, since it seemed I was often on a diet and tracking my calories. However, dieting was always an on again/off again thing with me, and I mostly thought I was controlling my calories, but looking back at it now, I can see that my weight gradually increased with each lunch that I ate.

Our company had cafeterias and lunch rooms in every building all over the place. There were plenty of food options and many of them were fattening. In my building, they even had a Krispy Kreme doughnut display right down the hall from the gym facility. Only I didn't eat the doughnuts.

Mostly I ate what was in my lunch bucket. I did have a problem with all the "friendly" food that was brought into the department for big meetings, and all those treats that other employees would set out, but I don't think that was mostly what MADE me fat. Those things helped KEEP me fat, but I think it was what I brought in my lunchbox that made me fat.

Now that I know WHAT WORKS, it is amazing to look back and see what DID NOT WORK. It's like my mother's mashed potatoes; I just ate and never realized that any one-particular food was worse for me, compared to other foods that I could have been eating.

Let me explain here, more about the lunches.

First, I bought stylish black square lunchboxes, one for my husband and one for me. I thought it would save money if we each brought all our food from home, and then ate only what we brought instead of buying expensive high-calorie food at work.

I cannot list here what my husband ate most days because he probably ate other foods during the day (and was also gaining a LOT of weight during that time, weight that he has since lost too), but below is what I usually ate:

My Breakfast - 430 Calories

2 slices bread—140 calories

4 Banquet turkey sausages—
(I put 2 sausages on a piece of bread
for a little sausage sandwich x 2)—
160 calories

1 banana—80 calories

Yogurt—mid morning snack—
60 calories

My Lunch–750 Calories

1 Pop-top can of soup–
200 calories per can

6-pak of cheese or peanut butter crackers–
220 calories

4-pak of cookies Chips Ahoy or Nutter Butter–
250 calories

1 fruit afternoon snack (apple, pear, etc.)–
80 calories

My Dinner and Evening Snack–500 Calories

Dinner for me at home was usually a Smart Ones–
300 calories

12-ounce package of frozen microwave vegetables–
100 calories

Fruit again or frozen yogurt for evening snack–
100 calories

Total around 1700 Daily Calories

Based on the above calculations, I ate **less than 1800 calories** per day.

So, if I normally only gain weight on more than 1800 calories a day, what happened to my weight? I should have been losing a little bit of weight each month, but I wasn't.

Apparently, I clearly didn't know what I was doing. To begin with, I didn't count any of the cream I put in my tea and coffee. In the morning, I usually drank two cups of coffee with a tablespoon or more of Coffeemate and I drank two or three cups of tea in the afternoon/evening with a couple of tablespoons of half-and-half in each.

If I added up all the Coffeemate and half-and-half calories in those hot drinks, I should add almost another 200 calories to my day. Also, I didn't count the tablespoon of light margarine that I put on my vegetables at dinner which is another 50 calories, so now my total was closer to **2000 Calories** each day.

That means that if I counted correctly, I should have gained weight, and I did, but that's not all I was eating. What about a couple of pretzel rods on a Wednesday evening, or maybe a couple pieces of pizza on a Friday evening? That all added up too, and I didn't always count those calories either. I guess I thought that if I didn't count them, that they didn't count.

Looking back though, it probably wasn't all the extra now-and-then foods that I ate, which did the most damage. It was because I was consistently eating around **500 more calories EVERY WORKDAY** in those go-packs of crackers and cookies in our lunchboxes, and my husband did the same thing. They added around 2500 calories each week for TEN or MORE YEARS!

What was I thinking?

Not only that, all those crackers and cookies were the wrong **KINDS** of foods to eat. All the sugar affected my metabolism, and those snacks all made me **HUNGRY,** instead of **SATISFIED**.

If I had only gained 5 pounds a year, in ten years, that adds up to 50 pounds right there.

I don't wonder anymore how I finally got to be more than 100 pounds overweight!!

CHAPTER SEVEN

....

BEGINNING MY JOURNEY TO BECOME LESS

A s I have gotten older, some of my health issues have resulted in me making more trips to the doctor, especially due to obesity. I now must take blood pressure and cholesterol medications, and as a result, I get regular blood tests to check on their effectiveness.

Through one of those blood tests, my doctor discovered that my A1C number was creeping up, and I was referred to an endocrinologist whom I see twice a year. When I started seeing this new doctor, I was at my highest weight ever, so he knew what bad shape I was in. He prescribed medication to help bring down my A1C number and to help keep me from becoming diabetic.

Diabetes is a big concern in my family since my maternal grandmother died in a diabetic coma when she was only forty years old. She had Type II diabetes, and her condition could have been treated if she had not been afraid to go to the doctor.

The year was 1946, and back in those days, doctors often practiced medicine out of their homes. My grandmother had been feeling ill and extremely thirsty, so my grandfather took her to the doctor. He waited for her in the car, and the story that I heard was that she knocked on the door, and when nobody answered, she came back to the car and told my grandfather that nobody was there, so they went back home.

It was the holiday season that year, and on Christmas evening, my mother was at her parents' house, and running a vacuum cleaner while her mother was napping in the next room. My mother was surprised that the noise from vacuuming didn't disturb her mother, so she checked in on her and couldn't wake her up.

The family rushed my grandmother to the hospital where she died that night. It was Christmas night 1946, and my grandmother never got to see her first granddaughter, because I wasn't born until almost two years later. I know that my grandmother could have had a much longer life, and I might have gotten to know her, if she had taken better care of her health.

Naturally, with my A1C numbers rising, my doctor warned me about my own risk of diabetes, and I was thankful that there was a medication that could help me.

I won't say the name of the medicine, but there are commercials on television all the time about A1C medications. You have probably seen the commercials, and your doctor will know about the medicines too. Most of the commercials, say that their product might help you lose a little weight "too".

After my doctor wrote the prescription, I picked it up on my way home that day, and I began taking my new medication the next day. Within a few days, something amazing happened to me. For the first time in my WHOLE LIFE I wasn't starving all the time. I still got hungry at mealtimes, but in the back of my mind, I wasn't thinking about food every minute of every day.

Over the next seven or eight months, I did lose 18-20 pounds, which was a good weight loss, but it was still somewhat "small" compared to my more than 120 pounds of excess weight. Just like the commercials had said, the medication "did help me to lose a little weight too".

What was most remarkable though, was the likely reason that I had lost the weight. This wasn't a diet drug, or something designed for weight loss, but by treating my A1C problem, it also diminished my CRAVING for food. I was mostly only hungry when it was close to a mealtime, and I wasn't still hungry after just eating a meal anymore.

Before that, except for maybe a big Thanksgiving dinner, I was almost never satisfied from eating a meal. For most of my life, I could always eat more, but now I could eat and not still be starving.

I came to realize that even back when I was a kid, and I wanted to steal my sister's milkshake at the "shaker counter", that it wasn't because I was hungry. It was probably because I was CRAVING, and she wasn't.

I don't know anything about insulin even now, but apparently something happened when I took the new medication. Maybe it corrected some condition that I had for years. What I always called "my tendency to gain weight" might have been something more. Maybe it was how my body processed insulin, and now this medication was setting straight something that always needed a correction. I don't know.

Until then, I never had any way to know that my life-long hunger might have really been a **compulsive craving and not hunger** at all.

I can't say know how this type of medicine would work for anyone else, but for me it was revolutionary. Even if I never lost another pound, it was a relief just to not be on the hunt in the kitchen for something to eat all the time.

I was finally able to sit and watch a TV show, and not be thinking in the back of my mind of what I would eat during the next commercial. Finally, a cup of tea was a complete snack. I didn't need a cookie, or pretzels or chips, or anything to quench my cravings.

Also, over those seven or eight months losing those 18-20 pounds, I wasn't doing anything to lose weight. At first, I didn't even realize that I was losing weight. After about a month, I got on the scale, and it seemed that I had lost three or four pounds. I didn't give it much thought. I was just taking my medication to bring down my A1C number. But I did notice that I wasn't starving all the time.

Because I was more than 100 pounds overweight, I was never excited about weighing myself, so I stayed off the scale most of the time. Years earlier, I had purchased a doctor's medical scale. It had the ruler at the top where you slide the weights across until the balance shows you your weight.

It was fairly depressing to get on that thing and see how fat I had become, and losing three or four pounds didn't enthuse me, but I decided to check on my weight every month or two, and I was noticing that my weight was creeping THE OTHER WAY now. It was creeping DOWN.

I didn't know why I was losing weight, but I must have been either eating less or my body was processing differently what I was eating, because I felt better when I ate, and I kept losing weight little by little.

Finally, after a few months, the downward weight trend ended at about 18-20 pounds lost, and even though my weight had stabilized, I continued having the additional benefit of NOT CRAVING anymore.

After getting accustomed to my new and improved lower weight, I had to face the fact that I still needed to lose much more, but I was not anxious to start another diet as I had in years past. I knew that the medication had changed the way I felt, and I didn't want to tinker with anything that might make the CRAVING begin again. For a while, I was content to just live in harmony with my still very-obese body.

After another six months, my life turned upside-down. We sold the house we had lived in for twenty years. We had bought a very small house to live in as retirees, and had years of clutter to pack up, give away or throw away. During all the stress and confusion of those days, my weight was the last thing on my mind.

I didn't think I was losing weight anymore, and my meals were mostly "hit-and-miss" during those hectic days. I even thought that I might be gaining back some weight.

To make matters even more confusing, the house where we were going wasn't available until a month after the house we were leaving got sold, so all our belongings had to be moved to storage while we waited for our next house to be vacant. This chaos was a "ready-made prescription" for someone like me to over-eat.

My husband and I had our own small trailer, and it took us about fifty trips to move all our smaller belongings to one or more of the five storage units that we had rented. By smaller belongings, I mean clothes, linens, dishes, bedding, and all the smaller furniture that we could carry. My medical scale was among one of the full-trailer trips that got stored, and I didn't see it again for a long time.

Finally, when the house was sold, the movers came on moving day, and took all the big furniture to the last of the empty storage units, and we took a couple wash baskets of our clothes and personal items to our daughter's house where we were staying for the month.

I didn't know what was happening with my weight during that month, and I wasn't thinking about it either.

On moving day, we had also packed up some of our important belongings into our van, along with what was in those wash baskets. We took only the baskets indoors, and we tried not to be underfoot with our daughter's family or take for granted their kind hospitality.

Finally, after the month ended, we got the keys to our then-vacant little retirement house and went over to see what needed to be done before we called to schedule the movers to bring our furniture back again.

It was a devastating shock when we walked through the doorway of our empty house, and the smell of cat urine hit us like a wet blanket. The prior residents must have had a hundred cats in there and no litter pans. We hadn't been in the house in a couple of years, and the folks living there seemed like nice clean people, but they apparently did not have any sense of smell.

I had to immediately call an air conditioning company to come out because the thermostat wire had been cut during the prior resident's move out, and the A/C wasn't working. It was the end of July and very hot, so I was thankful when the A/C guy soon arrived.

As we all stood out in the driveway, we could hear the A/C guy in there choking and gagging on the smell while he was trying to fix the air conditioning. During this chaos, my daughter arrived and saw me standing out there crying, and when she tried to enter the house, she backed out and said the house needed to be condemned. She said it wasn't safe to live there, and we would end up with respiratory problems if we slept there. Hearing that, I cried even harder.

I was thankful that the air conditioning was soon working, and I hoped the cool air would somehow mitigate the urine smell. Once the A/C guy left, the men went in and dragged out several large area rugs, and many smaller throw rugs, all of which were soaked with cat urine. Finally, we went back to our daughter's house not knowing what to do next.

What we did end up doing was to tear up every floor in the entire house. It was a small single-story house, but when we were finally done with that step, there was a dumpster full of urine-soaked flooring along with all the baseboards and other demolition debris.

We then had to paint every inch of underflooring with two coats of shellac paint to block the cat smell. It cost $600 for just the shellac. Then it cost $6,000 to have installers come in and install new Pergo flooring throughout the whole house.

Also, every single inch of walls and ceilings had to be washed and painted with two coats of paint. When we wiped the walls with a wet sponge, the sponge was covered with cat fur that was sticking to the walls in the dried moisture from the cat urine. You couldn't see the cat fur on the walls, but it was there. Also, all the lighting had to be taken down from the ceilings and washed because there was a sticky urine residue on all the glass and brass fixtures.

The kitchen was small, and there weren't many cupboards, but all the lower ones had to be torn out and replaced, because the cats had urinated down the front of the cabinets and you could see and smell the streaks of cat urine.

We ended up staying with our daughter for a couple of weeks until everything had been stripped out and thrown away, and the floors had been painted and the walls cleaned. Then we were able to bring in a couple of cots and a microwave so we could sleep there and work all day every day until we could get the place habitable again.

We could not move any of our furniture into the house from storage because it would all end up smelling like cat urine, and my husband was non-committal about ever living there at all since he has such a keen sense of smell. Even after everything was cleaned, painted, replaced, and made beautiful again, he would still get down on his hands and knees and sniff the corners of the floors to see if he could still smell cat "pee."

It took three whole months, before the house was finally and really-habitable, and we could get the movers to bring back our furniture. It cost more than $13,000 for the rehab project with us doing much of the work, plus another $3,000 in moving and storage expenses.

This was not the retirement experience I had worked my whole life hoping for, and under normal circumstances, it would have been "binging-made-to-order" for me, but somehow that wasn't what happened. I still wasn't craving and there wasn't much food around to eat anyway.

It was still summer, and each day one of us went to McDonalds and brought back large coffees and Egg McMuffins as we sat outside on lawn chairs and ate our breakfast before we got to work on the next project. For lunch and dinner, it was usually Smart Ones meals in the microwave, and there was always lots of diet soda and water to drink.

We ate off paper plates using plastic forks and spoons and drank out of paper cups that were left over from our morning McDonald's coffee. We were able to dig out the coffeemaker and a tea kettle from a storage unit, but it took months before I could locate my dishes and regular silverware.

So, that's mostly how and what we ate for those three months as we turned our house into a home again. After the initial demolition, the work was more tedious than hard, so it wasn't strenuous exercise. It was just us plodding along each day with a list of scrubbing, painting or whatever came next, until we could finally move in.

After the movers returned, and our things came back, I noticed my doctor's scale there in the pile of my reclaimed belongings, so I decided to hop on it to see what I weighed. I wore loose cotton shirts and twill capri pants throughout the rehab, so my clothes were already loose and not telling me what was happening with my weight.

I was still so fat, that a few pounds either way were hardly noticeable, so I was surprised to see that I had lost

another 20 pounds during that three months when I was
without a scale. I was relieved that I had not gained weight
with all the daily Egg McMuffins and coffee and whatever
else we were able to dig up to eat each day. I was thankful
that I had lost 20 more pounds and with the previous 20
pounds I had lost the year before, I was down a whole 40
pounds. While I was still 80 pounds overweight, I was relieved it wasn't more.

During all the chaos, I was still seeing the endocrinologist on a regular basis, and he was happy when I had lost
the first 20 pounds. On my next doctor appointment, he
was also surprised and pleased that I had lost another 20
pounds.

Since doctor appointments only last so long, it was
hard to explain to him what happened with the house rehab and how I lost the second 20 pounds. Besides he really wouldn't want to hear my sad story about the cat "pee"
and all that had happened. Anyway, he was happy I had
lost more weight, but of course I was still obese.

For almost the next whole year after the rehab project,
I never did anything else about my weight, and it didn't
seem to vary much from month to month. However, on
one later visit to the doctor, I saw that my weight was
suddenly up about six pounds, and I was concerned that
it might creep all the way back up. Still I wasn't craving
again, and I had never gone back to craving after I started
the A1C medication. But apparently, I was eating too much
because I had started to gain weight again.

Since I was alarmed about gaining back my weight, I told the doctor that I would really like to lose another 25 or 30 pounds, but I didn't know how I could do it.

I had lost the first 20 pounds just by taking the A1C medication which seemed to suppress my craving, and I lost the second 20 pounds by eating less throughout the rehab project.

I didn't have any other ideas about what to do to lose more weight except dieting, and exercise, but since I had unsuccessfully been that route dozens of times in my life, I decided to just leave it alone for then, and if possible, try not to gain back any more weight.

CHAPTER EIGHT

....

THE POWER OF *TRYING AGAIN*

I have heard that because Thomas Edison failed so many times trying to get the light bulb to work, that he once said, "I have not failed, I just found 10,000 ways that it won't work." I don't know if that is exactly what Thomas Edison said, but I know that is mostly what he did. I learned a lesson from Thomas Edison about never giving up, so trying one more time is what I finally did too.

My children were skinny kids growing up. They had to be because I was vigilant about their weight throughout their whole childhoods. Because of me being overweight as a child, I never wanted my kids to be overweight too, so I diligently monitored what they ate.

Now, I was never what one would call "mean" about food, and I never made my kids think they had to diet, but I was always careful about what and how much food I brought home, and how big the portions were at meals. Between meals, food was mostly off limits to them. The kids were permitted to eat a couple of cookies and a glass of milk for a snack, or maybe a small cupcake or a couple of pretzels. But they were never allowed to crunch through an entire bag of chips or pretzels or binge on other snacks.

The other thing that I regulated was the milk. We never had any milk in the house that wasn't skim. Before my first baby was six months old, he was already on his way to becoming a butterball because I had misunderstood the eating instructions from his pediatrician.

The baby was a robust little guy so the doctor thought I could start him on some solid food in the little jars of baby food from the supermarket. When the doctor told me to feed him his cereal, a fruit and a vegetable each meal along with his bottle, I thought he meant ALL THREE at each meal. I dutifully followed the instructions, and at the next three-month checkup, my nine-month old son was bursting out of his one-year-old baby clothes.

The doctor was shocked at his weight and when I told him what I had fed the baby, he said "No, not ALL of it at EVERY meal, just a bottle and a couple of tablespoons of ONE OF THEM at each meal." So already, I had to put my baby on a diet at less than a year old.

When I asked the doctor about the formula, I told him that I only drank instant powdered skim milk. He was pleased to know that, since he could see by my own size that I should be drinking skim milk. He told me that I could put skim milk in the baby's bottle instead of the formula. He said the instant milk was just as good as whole milk, so until my children were out of college, they drank powdered skim milk at home.

Of course, they were probably always drinking whole milk, and eating pizza and hamburgers and cake at school, since they bought their school lunches each day, but they never ate that way on a regular basis at home.

When they became adults, my kids were tall and lean. My son filled out a little more when he became a man, but my daughter was always a twig. That is why I was surprised one day when she told me that she had lost five pounds at Weight Watchers.

Through other means, I had lost about 40 pounds over eighteen months back a couple of years earlier, but I was still obese, and I seemed to be stuck there. I had asked my endocrinologist about losing another 25 or 30 pounds, and even though I tried to lose more weight, I was once again unsuccessful, but I was happy that I was still maintaining most of my 40-pound loss.

I had tried Weight Watchers many times throughout my life. Indeed, I could paper a room with all the weigh-in booklets, program books, and menu sheets that I had collected over the years. I still have a Rubbermaid tub full of them in the basement. But at the beginning of every year, I always dutifully signed up again for the Weight Watchers at Work program as part of my new year's resolution to lose weight.

Each year Weight Watchers always seemed to start a new-and-improved program with changes to their old program. As time went along, one thing I noticed was that they were adding more and different foods to their programs each year. It never seemed to matter what the new program was though. Whatever it was, it only worked for me for about a month when my weight would plateau. Then I soon would struggle to lose more weight, get discouraged, and then finally give up again.

I know they were always making improvements, but better food and more choices, made it harder for me to keep to my exchange or points limits. I used the slider cards, and the points calculator, whatever the latest program version was, trying to stay within the limits, and I was still always hungry. By then, I had mostly given up on Weight Watchers and thought of it as just another one of my many failures.

So now here I was, sitting at my daughter's place listening to this thin little twig tell me that she had just lost five pounds at Weight Watchers. I must have stared at her for a whole minute before I could think of something to say. Finally, I had to ask her if she *really* meant that she had lost five pounds at Weight Watchers. I asked her if she really had five pounds that she needed to lose. I asked her where she went to meetings. I was astonished.

I could hardly believe that Weight Watchers had a program that was effective enough to help someone as fit as my daughter lose five pounds. She told me that she had signed up for the on-line Weight Watchers APP, and that it had really helped her to figure out what she was eating and what she should be eating, and that it was easy to lose the five pounds.

I had a dozen questions about Weight Watchers that day, and what most intrigued me was that if someone lean like my daughter could lose weight there, then maybe I could lose weight there after all. My daughter told me that there were 200 free foods that I could eat any time I was hungry, and she showed me the list that was out there on the internet somewhere. I thought that it must be a different program than they ever had before, and if it really worked, I wanted in on it too.

While I sat there that afternoon, my daughter helped me to sign in and register for the Weight Watchers Meetings program. Then the next day she came to our house and helped her dad register for the on-line Weight Watchers APP like the one she used.

My husband is six feet tall and he weighed about 200 pounds most of his adult life. In his fifties he added probably another 20 pounds due to a slower life-style and from eating foods that I packed in his lunchbox. His weight mostly stayed at around 220 pounds for the next ten years.

Later he had some health issues and he was prescribed medications that helped his weight zoom up to almost 280 pounds. Now after Weight Watchers, his weight is down again to 225 pounds, but until that day, given my own many failures at trying to lose my own weight, I couldn't imagine how to help him lose all his weight too.

On that day, our daughter gave us hope that here was finally something that could help us to lose some weight and maybe get healthier.

After signing up for Weight Watchers, it was a couple of days before I attended my first meeting, and I already began to have doubts that it would work for me. I had signed up for six months of meetings though, so I realized that even if it didn't work, I was stuck for a while.

I looked up locations and times where I could attend meetings, and I discovered that the best meeting location for me was in the little town I had moved away from, back when I sold the house. A couple of days later I showed up bright and early for my first Weight Watchers meeting since I had last quit the Weight Watchers at Work program.

I wasn't surprised by the high weight number that registered when I stepped on the scale, since I had already weighed myself on my doctors' scale at home. I was still easily 80 pounds overweight, and this was my lowest Weight Watchers weight in years.

I was surprised by how many members filed in as I sat there reading the materials that I had been given. I arrived there half an hour early and I was the first person on the scale, but by the time the meeting started, there must have been fifty people there.

The meeting leader was cheerful and upbeat, and as I sat and listened to the topic of the week, my first impression of her was that she was perky and cute. She looked really thin and really young, and I wondered if she could truly understand what it felt like to be old and fat like me.

I sat there thinking back to when I had reached my Weight Watchers goal weight years before. I was in my mid 30's, which was more than thirty years ago, and I remembered my leader from back then. She was in her early 50's at the time and she was very mature and maybe even a little harsh. Her very-disciplined manner always kept me on my toes.

As this new leader covered the topic of the week, and asked for participation, the group seemed to be highly-engaged and was responding well to her energy. Everyone seemed to be having fun and joining in, but I began to feel a bit like an outcast. The meeting seemed more like a social than a class, and since I am an introvert and not very friendly, I felt out of place.

As the meeting continued, and everyone was sharing and asking questions, I had begun looking up other meeting times and locations on my phone, to see if there was something else where I could find maybe an older leader who had had a really-big weight problem like mine. I abandoned my search when the meeting ended, and it was time for me to stay for orientation.

There were a few of us new members there that day, and after we herded together, the leader began covering the program handbook for us. She also explained the free-foods list, and I was still surprised at the large amount of food that I would be able to eat. I remembered in the past, when more and better foods were added to the program, how hard it was for me to stay within my points limits, and I thought it would be just another disappointing weight-loss experience to add to my long list of failures.

I didn't believe I could lose weight eating so much of all those free foods, so finally I piped up and asked her if she really believed that I could eat that way and still lose weight. She assured me that I could and that I would, an

answer that annoyed me and made me even more skeptical. Finally, I sniveled back at her that I didn't think it was
possible to lose weight eating so much free food, and then
I asked her just how much weight she had lost anyway.

As she warmly smiled at me and said just four small
words, "over two hundred pounds", I was stunned into
silence. Here I was being a rude and pompous know-it-all,
and here she was being kind, helpful, and cheerful, and
with just those four small words, she graciously called
check-mate on me.

What could I say? Eating all that food must work. Here
was living proof of that fact. Anyone should have been
thrilled about the possibility, and while I was still a bit
skeptical, from that moment on, I got on board.

I did ask her why she didn't announce her weight loss
at the beginning of the meeting and pass around her "before and after pictures". That was a routine that was done
in every meeting I had ever attended all those years before. Also, that would have kept me from searching for
another meeting as I sat there that day.

She said that they didn't do that anymore, but she
wouldn't say why. Later, I gathered from things I heard at
meetings, that some members could be offended by the
pictures, maybe they even felt fat shamed if they were not
having good losses that week themselves.

I don't know if that's true, but I think it's a big mistake
to hide the successes of Weight Watchers members. Even
if I am having a bad day, the success of others helps to
motivate me. It gives me faith that if you can lose all that

weight following this program, then I can lose weight too. It's really an inspiration and after hearing about her weight loss, I was inspired.

CHAPTER NINE

....

THE ANSWER I WAITED FOR MY WHOLE LIFE

So how did I lose 100 pounds? What exactly did I do? For starters, I cannot publish the Weight Watchers program for you here in my book nor do I want to. I do not represent Weight Watchers and I receive NO BENEFIT whatsoever for any positive statements that I make or have made regarding their weight-loss program.

My story is not about Weight Watchers anyway. My story is about my fat life and *How I Lost 100 Pounds at Age 70*. Throughout the years, Weight Watchers was part of my life many times, so of course I cannot help but to include my Weight Watchers story here in my book. However, it wasn't following the Weight Watchers program alone that brought about my amazing weight loss. There is much more to it than that.

It took me seventy years to finally learn how to lose 100 pounds, and in those years, I probably lost and re-gained 100 pounds many times, in smaller losses, over-

and-over again, but somehow those pounds always returned.

But finally, this time was different!

It seems strange to be saying that because when we
start a new diet, isn't that what we *always* say? And the
story always ends the same. We lose weight, we gain it
back, and soon we are fatter than ever.

But for me, this time really **WAS** different.

Why was this time different?

To begin with, my doctors, Weight Watchers, Jenny
Craig, even Dr. Oz, always seemed to be telling me the
same thing. It is something so basic that I probably should
have realized it back at the grapefruit diet, and maybe even
back at the "shaker counter".

The message that everyone seemed to be sending to
me my whole life, a message that I probably heard a hundred times, was that I needed to eat the *RIGHT* **FOODS**.

The problem though was that while I **heard** it before,
I never *believed* it before. But this time, I **heard** it and *I*
finally believed it.

What they each seemed to be saying in their own different words was, **ALL CALORIES ARE NOT THE
SAME!**

Because of that, not only should I eat the **RIGHT
FOODS**, but if I do, I can eat **MORE** of them, *and that
was the answer to my life-long weight problem* .

I don't need to be hungry anymore!!!

Throughout my entire fat life, I have been counting
calories, and no matter how many times they added up to

1400, I still couldn't lose the weight. I was eating less and starving more, but never losing the weight. And even though I was always told to eat the right foods, I apparently never really understood what the right foods were, nor did I understand that the right foods could be **WONDERFUL** foods.

It might have been because of my mother's enormous bowls of mashed potatoes, or those fried potato patties, and fried chicken. Maybe it was the two-layer cakes with all the icing in between the layers and piled high on top. Whatever it was, I always thought the key to losing weight was **EATING LESS,** and that was something I couldn't do for very long.

What I finally learned this time is that the **KEY** to losing weight is **EATING MORE.**

The KEY to my amazing weight loss at the age of seventy is that I finally learned that to NEVER BE FAT AGAIN, meant that I needed to **STOP BEING SO HUNGRY ALL THE TIME!!**

It sounds weird, but it's true.

The reason diets never worked for me was *that I couldn't stay hungry enough, long enough, to lose enough©.* Instead, what I should have done was to eat **ENOUGH** of the **RIGHT FOODS** so that I wouldn't want or need to eat the wrong foods.

In all my past dieting, I was always hungry, starving even. I always had to count my daily calories, or my exchanges, or my points, and when I ran out of them each day, usually by lunch time, I had to starve for the remainder of the day, until my next-day allotment of them rolled around at breakfast. That never worked because I got too hungry and then gave up.

The secret was, that I needed **MORE FOOD**, and more of the *RIGHT FOOD*.

So, what does that mean? What is the right food? What exactly do I eat now?

To begin with, I used the free-food list. I live and breathe by it. Even at my Weight Watchers meetings, when anyone asks me how I lost my weight, my response is always the same two words, "Free Food." I think even they might be getting tired of hearing me say it.

Remember, that day at my daughter's, even before I joined Weight Watchers, I read the free-food list on the internet. It's out there for everyone to read, so it's no secret. It's probably a similar list that any doctor would give to someone trying to lose weight.

There are foods on that list like eggs, and fish, and skinless chicken breast, and vegetables, such as most kinds of beans, and most other vegetables too. Even corn and peas are there, and there have always been fruits, but now even bananas are free foods.

Back in the old days many of those foods were limited, a cup here, a half-a-cup there, or maybe eat something just twice a week, and almost everything needed to be tracked. But now, I could eat more of the foods on that list whenever, and as often as I want, and free foods never need to be tracked!

That meant that I could eat a couple of hard-boil eggs for a snack, or if I had a taste for something sweet, could have a banana in the evening, even if I already had one at breakfast. In the evening, or anytime, I could microwave a bowl of pinto beans, and pile on some salsa, and stir in a slice of Velveeta cheese (which happens to have a small 1-point value), and I would have a warm, tasty and filling snack.

No more potato chips for me either. If I sometimes get a hunger for some carbs, I can microwave an entire 12-oz bag of frozen corn and sprinkle on some salt, and then add in a teaspoon of light margarine (again a small 1-point value), and I can sit there and eat that whole bowl of corn, and STILL LOSE WEIGHT!!

Remember my obstetrician who once said that "corn was for slopping hogs". Like I said before, HE WAS WRONG! Corn is for *losing weight*.

Somewhere along the way, somebody realized that there are lots of great foods that fill us up and that we can eat and still lose weight. No more eating celery, and carrot sticks, until we finally reach for that bag of pretzels or that package of cookies.

My husband is a "sweets junkie", so there are always three or four sweet snacks that we have on hand that he eats and loves. In the fridge, we always have a large container of sugar-free Jello along with a carton of cool-whip. Cool-whip is one of those foods that need to be tracked, but again, it's only 1 point (out of my 23 daily points).

Also, we keep canned (zero-points) fruit cocktail on hand, which is terrific too with a tablespoon of cool-whip. There are sugar-free cake mixes out there that I bake into big chocolate cupcakes. I keep the baked cupcakes in the freezer in a zip lock bag, and my husband can quickly defrost one any time. The cupcakes track at 3 or 4 points, but again, with a couple tablespoons of cool whip on top, there is no need for junky cookies for him.

He would tell you that he has never eaten so well in all the years we've been married, and he has lost more than 50 pounds at the same time he has been eating MORE and BETTER FOOD.

Now it is always possible that I could gorge myself on all the free foods, and not lose weight or maybe even gain weight that week. But that is not what happens, at least not for me.

Remember back when I challenged my Weight Watchers leader during my orientation about not believing that I could eat all those foods and still lose weight?

Well she said something interesting then. She said that after a few weeks, I would learn when I had eaten enough to be satisfied, and if I really ate too much, that it would show up at the scale. Then I could adjust my amounts or try some other free foods instead. But she assured me that I would not need to go hungry while I lost weight, and she was right.

The foods I am eating now are substantial enough, and are satisfying enough, that I am not running to the refrigerator during every commercial to look for something to binge on. I know however, that if I am hungry, that I CAN RUN to the refrigerator and will find something to eat that I love and that won't make me fat. How wonderful is that!

By now, I understand enough about what to eat and how to eat, that I could probably go on alone, but I will always be a Weight Watcher. While I don't promote Weight Watchers, I feel free to say good things about them, because they have the program and the tools that work. After all my tries at losing weight, I found that they have almost perfected their program, so I hope they won't change it from what works!!

They did change their name last year to WW, but they will always be Weight Watchers to me. They have great people, as well as great tools that make it easy for me to know what to eat. Their phone APP has a tracking tool for clicking in the foods that do need to be tracked. You can eat really anything you want, just track the foods that are NOT free foods; breads, pasta, anything. There are no forbidden foods.

Also, in their APP is a handy little icon that brings up a scanning box that lets you easily scan a UPC bar code. You can scan practically any bar code on any food package and the APP will tell you the points per serving value of the food.

One day, I spent about two hours at Walmart, scanning hundreds of foods looking for anything that was zero or low in points, and I made my own free-foods grocery shopping list so that I would know what to buy each time.

Again, I am not telling you to join WW. I am just saying what I did. Of course, anyone can follow the free-foods list and find much of the RIGHT FOOD, on their own, right there on the internet.

However, there are lots of foods not on that list that all of us eat all the time, and I can't tell you an easier way to know what and how much of those foods to eat than to just join the program. The phone APP was all that my husband needed, and it is not expensive.

You might want to do something different than WW, and if so, you can probably get similar information from your doctor, or maybe at the gym. You may want to try losing weight other ways like I did over the years. These days, there are many diet books out there, with lots of weight loss ideas, and maybe some of those will work for you.

But for me and **MY** fat life (and how I lost 100 pounds at the age of 70), WW was high on the list of things that helped me accomplish that incredible achievement.

There is ONE OTHER THING THAT I DID to lose 100 pounds that needs more than a mention here.

I took all the TIME I NEEDED to lose my weight.

TIME is a deciding factor for success. We need to give ourselves enough time to accomplish anything in life. When it comes to weight-loss, if you aren't starving yourself all the time, and you are eating all the food you need to be satisfied and healthy, you won't feel rushed and in a hurry. You will be amazed to see those pounds melt away as you lose weight a little at a time, and over time, you can achieve your own success.

I plan to keep on doing the same thing for the rest of my life. For me, it is so **EASY** because **I am NOT DIET-ING or STARVING** anymore!!!

You will remember that I said that the reason that diets never worked for me, was *that I couldn't stay hungry enough, long enough, to lose enough*©.

When I finally started eating enough of the **RIGHT FOODS**, I began losing weight slow and steady. The reason that worked so well for me, was that *I could go* slow and steady, since *I NEVER HAD TO GO HUNGRY TOO!*

I wanted to lose an average of a pound a week and I did even better. I averaged five pounds each month without much effort and even **WITHOUT EXERCISING**.

To ensure I was getting accurate weight numbers, I usually ate light the day before my weigh-ins. I didn't want to bulk up on pinto beans, or corn, or lots of bananas or even lots of salt the day before my weigh-in. I always got weighed in the morning before eating or drinking anything. While I drink two or three 16 oz bottles of water a day, nobody wants to drink a bottle of water on the way to the scale and have it become part of a weigh-in number. I always wear the same clothes too.

Small weight losses can be camouflaged with bulk food and water, but real weight loss stays with you from week to week. There were weeks that I lost a pound or even two, and weeks when I only lost six-tenths of a pound.

But when I added them all up, they turned into 5, and 10, and 25, and 50 pounds and up.

Our daughter calls us her *amazing* shrinking parents and she is right. Losing 100 pounds at the age of 70 is *amazing*. And what is even more *amazing* is that now I know that I can eat this way for the rest of my life, and

I NEVER **NEED** TO BE FAT ANYMORE!!!

....

CHAPTER TEN

BEHAVIORS WEIGHT LOSS FORMULA

VKB-Behaviors-Weight-Loss-Formula

$$(G=(W+T+A)>H) \text{ ©}$$

(Goal = (Willpower + Time + Accountability) > Hunger) ©

This is just a little something extra to help you visualize how your behaviors can affect your success or failure at losing weight.

It might seem unusual to even find a formula in a "How-I-Lost-Weight" book, but this formula might help explain why it's often such a struggle to lose that weight. In my case, I recognized patterns of behavior in my own lifetime of dieting, and when I examined what I did in trying to lose weight, I applied my own behavior to this formula to help me figure it out. Of course, this formula is behavioral rather than scientific, but it might explain the effect of our behaviors versus our often-unsatisfactory dieting results.

We eat calories (energy), and we mostly cannot change what our bodies do with them. If 500 calories of zucchini, and 500 calories of chocolate cake are each burned in a laboratory setting such as in test tubes (in an isolated system), they will each release the same amount of energy.

But that is not what happens when we put those same foods into our bodies. Our bodies might either burn them, store them, do some of each, or do something else altogether. Also, the next time we consume those same foods, they may store and burn differently than the last time. This might be one reason why there is no real fool-proof or easy formula for losing weight.

So, we know that we cannot control what happens to the food we have eaten. What do we control then, or better yet WHAT CAN WE CONTROL?

The answer is **OUR BEHAVIOR**.

And by controlling our behavior we can PLAN to SUCCEED!

Losing 100 pounds was an amazing achievement for me especially at my age, and I wanted to understand what happened this time that was different. In evaluating all my successes and all my failures through all those many years of struggle, I finally saw the patterns of what I did and what I did not do.

When I looked at all the pieces of my weight-loss puzzle, I realized that for me, there was a simple formula to help explain why I kept failing over-and-over again. Almost every time, I had planned for failure, and I always succeeded at failing.

This formula is only intended as a template for testing out behaviors. The components of the formula are explained on the following pages.

VKB-Behaviors-Weight-Loss-Formula

$$(G=(W+T+A)>H) \text{ ©}$$

(Goal = (Willpower + Time + Accountability) > Hunger) ©

What I finally learned was that H (Hunger) was the determining factor in my success or failure at weight loss.

In losing or maintaining weight, all my behavior factors had to outweigh the value of H (Hunger). If H was greater than all (or in some cases any) of my other behavior factors, then I would once again fail. I rate each factor as either LOW or HIGH except H which is on a 1-10 scale. Below are explanations of the Factors:

1. GOAL in this formula is defined as the pounds lost, or the low weight or the low weight range that you must achieve to consider yourself successful when you consistently weigh yourself on an accurate standard scale.

2. WILLPOWER is defined as what you are WILL-ING to DO to both reach and maintain your goal weight. When we think of willpower, we usually think of "going hungry to lose weight", but it is more than that. Willpower should include compo-

nents like cost, effort, food, satisfaction, and desire. Willpower is **WILLINGNESS**. You must be willing to do what works to reach your goal. You can define willpower in different ways using this list of willpower components or even by adding your own.

Willpower Component Examples:

    a. Cost – You are willing to spend money to join Weight Watchers or to pay for a trainer, or to spend $500 dollars a month for mail-order or other special food.

    b. Effort – You are willing to attend meetings or to walk three miles a day, or even ten miles a day, or you are willing to try cooking some recipes from lite-eating cookbooks, or you are willing to go to the gym three days a week. Also, you are willing to track your food to document your pattern of eating the right foods.

    c. Food – You will eat better foods. While you used to eat lots of red meat, and sugary treats, you are now willing to eat more chicken and fish, and you are willing to dine out less often.

    d. Satisfaction – You really enjoyed the foods you ate before, and you enjoyed eating later, and eating sweets. You enjoyed special beverages and parties. You are willing to sacrifice some of your satisfaction to achieve your goal.

e. Desire – For some people their desire to reach goal is so strong that they practically starve themselves, for others they are only dieting because their doctors advised them to lose weight.

3. TIME is defined as the number of days, months and even years that you are willing to spend on the changes you make to achieve your goals.

4. ACCOUNTABILITY is defined as getting weighed on a regular basis. You will track your weight-loss journey by getting weighed at weight-loss meetings, or getting weighed by your trainer, or at your gym. If you are unwilling to have someone weigh and track your progress, your commitment to weight loss may slide. If you gain weight, you will recommit to food tracking to ensure that you are eating enough of the right foods.

5. HUNGER is defined as the amount of discomfort you are willing to endure to lose weight. It is common to be asked at the doctor's office, to "rate your pain today on a scale of 1-10". If you tell the nurse that your pain is a 1 or 2, nobody is very

concerned, but if you report an 8 or 9, the doctor will want to investigate further.

By the same standard, you should rate your hunger on a daily (even hourly) basis using the same scale of 1-10. To be successful at losing or maintaining your weight, you will want to keep your hunger level low most of the time. At high hunger levels, you will not want anyone to stand between you and the refrigerator. That is a formula for failure.

SO HOW DOES THIS FORMULA WORK?

It's a very simple and basic formula. You can use it to group all your weight-loss behaviors into one of the four factors to determine why you succeeded or failed, or to predict future success or failure. Even before you begin, if you score each factor, you will have some idea of your outcome as the factors will help you determine your likely goal score.

EXAMPLE of MY GOAL:

I wanted to reach my weight loss goal, at an average of ONE pound a week for as long as it took.

FORMULA RESULT from Factors Below:

(Goal	(Willpower	Time	Accountability)	Hunger)
=	+	+	>	
Reached	High	High	High	2

WILLPOWER was HIGH because I was willing to invest in the cost of Weight Watchers meetings, make the

effort to track food and attend meetings, shop for and prepare food that was low in points and high in satisfaction,
and I had a desire to finally conquer my obesity to improve my health and satisfy the concerns of my doctors.

TIME was HIGH because there was plenty of it or at
least as long as it takes. Since there was no fixed time and
no fixed deadline, I was able to take all the time I needed
to figure out the RIGHT foods to eat and learn how best
to prepare them.

ACCOUNTABILITY was HIGH because I attended
Weight Watchers meetings often and had regular recorded weigh-ins and encouragement from the staff and
my Weight Watcher leader.

HUNGER was LOW because I was eating my daily
points along with as much free food as I wanted and
needed to keep from being hungry. I kept my hunger
level rating at 1-3 most of the time, and never let it go to
the level of 8 or 9 or 10. If I sensed that I was getting
hungry, I ate a banana, or a hard-boiled egg, or some other
free food that satisfied my hunger. I know that hunger is
not my weight-loss friend anymore but my weight-loss
enemy.

EXAMPLE 1 GOAL:

You are going to your 10-year reunion in 8 weeks and you want to lose 30 pounds.

FORMULA RESULT from Factors Below:

(Goal	(Willpower	Time	Accountability)	Hunger)
=	+	+	>	
Likely Miss	High	Low	High	8

WILLPOWER is HIGH because your desire is high, and you are anxious to lose weight. You are willing to exercise and to practically "fast" to help reach your goal. However, you are likely to miss your goal because you will be too hungry from eating less food, and too worn out from your excessive effort in exercising.

TIME is LOW because you have a short and fixed deadline. You must lose 3.75 pounds in each of the next 8 weeks. It is possible, but it may not be enough time to reach goal.

ACCOUNTABILITY is HIGH because your husband will weigh you each week, and you will know your progress.

HUNGER is also HIGH because you will eat less food to lose more weight faster. Because the Hunger component is HIGH from virtual fasting in trying to reach your goal in such a short time, you should plan to score your goal as "Likely Miss".

EXAMPLE 2 GOAL:

You are going to need back surgery, but your surgeon wants you to lose 20 pounds before setting a date. Your back is uncomfortable, but there is no fixed deadline:

FORMULA RESULT from Factors Below:

(Goal	(Willpower	Time	Accountability)	Hunger)
=	+	+	>	
Likely Reach	High	High	High	3

WILLPOWER is HIGH because you are uncomfortable and you want to get your surgery over and done with, but you are not desperate. You are willing to make the effort to cook and eat different and better food choices.

TIME is HIGH because there is plenty of it since there is no fixed deadline for the surgery. Even if you only lose 4 pounds a month, you should be able to reach your goal in less than six months.

ACCOUNTABILITY is HIGH because you will get weighed at your monthly doctor check-ups, and you and he will both know your progress (even better if you can get weighed more often).

HUNGER is LOW because you can eat more food over a longer time-period and still lose weight. You will not be starving and will likely stay with your eating program.

SUMMARY OF FORMULA:

As you can see by the formula examples, the higher your Willpower, Time, and Accountability Factors are compared to your Hunger Factor, the more likely you are to lose weight and keep it off.

Also, by prototyping your plan for losing weight against this formula, you can "story-board" your likelihood of success or failure. Instead of jumping into a quick-weight-loss diet and feeling like a failure later, you will be able to see from the start that you are sabotaging your efforts by not allowing enough of the first three Factors to overcome the H Factor.

While the formula is just a simple subjective guide as to how to think about our weight-loss behaviors, I found that all the examples of my previous attempts to lose weight, when plotted against the formula, have revealed many of the pitfalls that contributed to my past failures.

On the following pages are three blank formula worksheets to use in helping you pencil in your own plan to modify your behaviors in achieving your own weight-loss success.

YOUR PERSONAL GOAL WORKSHEET #1

Describe the Goal You are Trying to Reach:

_____

_____

_____

_____

_____

NOTE: Evaluating your expected behaviors before beginning, will help you to define your plan for success.

FORMULA RESULT – Based on the Factors you describe below, select either Reach, Likely Reach, Likely Miss, or Miss in the grid box below under "Goal".

(Goal	(Willpower	Time	Accountability)	Hunger)
=	+	+	>	

WILLPOWER Factor – Rate your Willpower as High or Low in the above grid box based on what you are "willing" to do to reach your goal as you describe below:

_____

_____

_____

_____

_____

TIME Factor – Rate your Time as High or Low in the above grid box based on the amount of time as your time-line to reach goal as you describe below:

_____

_____

_____

_____

_____

ACCOUNTABILITY Factor – Rate your Accountability as High or Low in the above grid box based on your planned weigh-ins and who will be weighing you as you describe below:

_____

_____

_____

_____

_____

HUNGER Factor – Rate your Hunger on a scale of 1-10 on how hungry you plan to be in the above grid box. Describe below why you chose this Hunger level (the other three factors will impact how hungry you will often be) as you describe below:

_____

_____

_____

_____

_____

YOUR PERSONAL GOAL WORKSHEET #2

Describe the Goal You are Trying to Reach:

_____

_____

_____

_____

_____

NOTE: Evaluating your expected behaviors before beginning, will help you to define your plan for success.

FORMULA RESULT – Based on the Factors you describe below, select either Reach, Likely Reach, Likely Miss, or Miss in the grid box below under "Goal".

(Goal	(Willpower	Time	Accountability)	Hunger)
=	+	+	>	

WILLPOWER Factor – Rate your Willpower as High or Low in the above grid box based on what you are "willing" to do to reach your goal as you describe below:

_____

_____

_____

_____

_____

TIME Factor – Rate your Time as High or Low in the above grid box based on the amount of time as your timeline to reach goal as you describe below:

_____
_____
_____
_____
_____

ACCOUNTABILITY Factor – Rate your Accountability as High or Low in the above grid box based on your planned weigh-ins and who will be weighing you as you describe below:

_____
_____
_____
_____
_____

HUNGER Factor – Rate your Hunger on a scale of 1-10 on how hungry you plan to be in the above grid box. Describe below why you chose this Hunger level (the other three factors will impact how hungry you will often be) as you describe below:

_____
_____
_____
_____
_____

YOUR PERSONAL GOAL WORKSHEET #3

Describe the Goal You are Trying to Reach:

_____

_____

_____

_____

NOTE: Evaluating your expected behaviors before beginning, will help you to define your plan for success.

FORMULA RESULT – Based on the Factors you describe below, select either Reach, Likely Reach, Likely Miss, or Miss in the grid box below under "Goal".

(Goal	(Willpower	Time	Accountability)	Hunger)
=	+	+	>	

WILLPOWER Factor – Rate your Willpower as High or Low in the above grid box based on what you are "willing" to do to reach your goal as you describe below:

_____

_____

_____

_____

_____

TIME Factor – Rate your Time as High or Low in the above grid box based on the amount of time as your time-line to reach goal as you describe below:

_____

_____

_____

_____

_____

ACCOUNTABILITY Factor – Rate your Accountability as High or Low in the above grid box based on your planned weigh-ins and who will be weighing you as you describe below:

_____

_____

_____

_____

_____

HUNGER Factor – Rate your Hunger on a scale of 1-10 on how hungry you plan to be in the above grid box. Describe below why you chose this Hunger level (the other three factors will impact how hungry you will often be) as you describe below:

_____

_____

_____

_____

_____

ABOUT THE AUTHOR

This creative author grew up in a challenging and scary world. She learned early that her life would require faith and courage to survive and to overcome life's obstacles. Over the years, she reached many milestones in her own life including teaching college, writing for a large city newspaper, and providing analytical support to multiple major corporations. Her books "No Ashes for Me", "Dos and Don'ts when You've Been Dumped", and "Nobody NEEDS to be FAT Anymore", are written as helpful resources designed to inspire her readers in overcoming their own life's challenges and in reaching toward their own happiness and satisfaction.